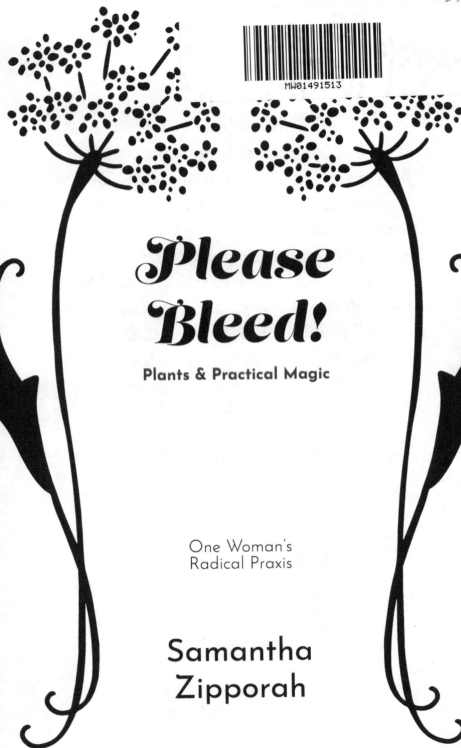

MW01491513

Please Bleed!

Plants & Practical Magic

One Woman's
Radical Praxis

Samantha
Zipporah

"*I am my own healer. I have a radiant voice within that guides me. I can make decisions for myself. I can rely on others as needed, but at my discretion. It is my body, my health, my balance, & my responsibility to make right choices for myself. Right choices include working with competent health-care professionals when necessary, allowing friends & family to help as needed, &, above all, being true to my beliefs, with the wisdom & willingness to change as part of the path of healing.*"

Rosemary Gladstar

Acknowledgements & Source Materials

There is nothing new under the sun. I stand on the shoulders of giantesses. These are just a few of the wells I have been blessed to draw from.

People

Casandra Johns houseofhands.net

Molly Dutton Kenny mollyduttonkenny.com

Alex Svoboda arisebotanicals.com

Ellie Mae Mitchell @moonbowmedicinals

Kelsey Jae kelseyjae.com

Megan Alton meganalton.com

Source Material

Wise Woman Herbal For The Childbearing Year by Susun Weed

Sisterzeus.com

Natural Liberty by Sage Femme Collective

Robin Rose Bennet's informal QAL study

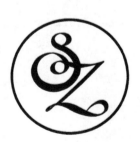

ISBN 978-1-63760-395-6

Preface

The information found in "Please Bleed!" will only be practically (rather than theoretically) useful if the reader knows

* **AT LEAST**
  the expected timing of their normal menstruation,

  or

* **AT BEST**
  the timing of their fertile window, ovulation,
  & "oops" sperm exposure

If the reader is aware of the timing of their expected menstruation, the information found in "Please Bleed!" may be used with the intention to help stimulate menstruation

* *After* an "Oops!"

* *Before* a period has been missed

The herbal options presented in "Please Bleed!" are not meant to be used regularly as a method of contraception, nor are they intended to be used to stimulate abortion after a period has been missed.

Ideally, the reader will take in this information during a non-emergent state & consider thoughtfully how best to integrate it into their own unique Conscious Contraception practice. This work can help one formulate a "Plan B" for avoiding pregnancy when a "Plan A" of avoiding sperm exposure during the fertile window fails.

The content in "Please Bleed!" primarily consists of excerpts from a more robust offering, The Conscious Contraception Skillshare, which is (likely, depending on when you're reading this!) available on my website www.samanthazipporah.com. The Conscious Contraception Skillshare provides instruction for the practice of the sympto-thermal method of fertility awareness as a method of contraception. Along with the basic data & skills needed to practice fertility awareness, the Conscious Contraception Skillshare includes extensive information & inspiration for healing & cultivating awareness of the menstrual cycle, our sexual power, & spiritual connection to our erotic life force.

I have created "Please Bleed!" as a shorter, more accessible source of education for folks not ready or able to take the deep dive into the whole of the Conscious Contraception Skillshare.

"Please Bleed!" is meant to inform, not instruct.

The information you'll find here will be most readily applicable for those who are already familiar or competent with tracking their cycle, & those who have some experience working with plant medicine.

Disclaimer

I am not your authority.

I am not a professional or certified herbalist, fertility awareness instructor, or healthcare provider. I am an ally & an educator. I'm a citizen scientist, an anarchist, & a witch. My offerings are meant to facilitate soulful embodiment, radical self awareness, & meaningful self determination. My work is not meant to replace your critical thinking skills, intuition, or support from other skilled healers.

Any & all recommendations herein are not prescriptions, guarantees, or diagnoses; they are for informational purposes only.

Gender Inclusivity

An individual's reproductive organs do not define their sexual preference or gender. All of our bodies came out of a womb. Knowledge about & care for their function is vital for all individual identities, & our collective culture as a whole.

I strive to make my work accessible & inclusive for diverse identities by referring to specific body parts & physiologic processes without assuming the gender or sexual preference of the person to whom the body or process belongs.

Trauma Informed

A tragically large number of us with wombs & vaginas have experienced some kind of physical or sexual violence. Even if we have not experienced physical abuse or assault, the dominant culture's treatment of our sexuality & fertility is psychologically, spiritually, & emotionally abusive. Many of us experience things like dissociation & depersonalization with our bodies & their functions as a result of generations of trauma, abuse, & being disconnected from our agency.

Practicing cycle awareness, feeling one's cervix, or tracking one's nuanced inner experience while imbibing plant medicines can be challenging or even impossible because of past traumas. I mention this here not to discourage individuals from gaining skills for embodiment & acheiving body literacy, but to encourage folks to be incredibly gentle, patient, & kind with themselves wherever they are in their process of inhabiting their bodies. Most importantly, I encourage everyone to seek support from healing artists & allies who can guide us into greater feelings of safety & self awareness.

"Please Bleed" is written in a voice speaking to the individual whose sperm exposure was by (hopefully happy, loving) accident, not by violence. While plants & practical magic can support us after sexual assault also, I strongly encourage safe human council & care rather than a DIY approach to healing & integration in the case of sexual violence.

Contents

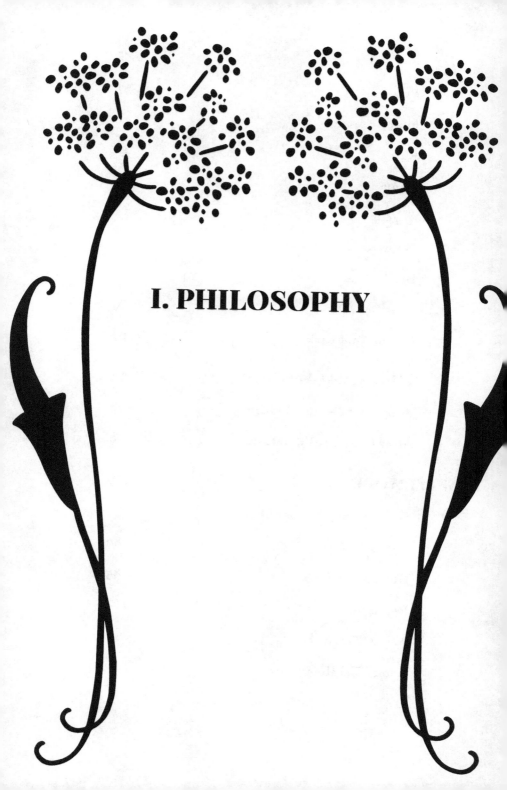

I. PHILOSOPHY

**"Herbal education begins
with changing our consciousness."**

Pam Montgomery

Why learn about herbal fertility management?

I have listened to many comrades make statements like "We must learn herbal (or home) abortion methods to protect ourselves from our fascist government's oppression!" or "We must learn how to avoid pregnancy in case the government takes away our access to clinical options (pills, IUDs, patches, etc)!"

While these statements have validity, they do not illustrate my personal motivation for learning about how to manage my fertility without asking anyone for permission, or consuming from industries that do not share my ethics.

To me, radical, DIY, community supported, non clinical fertility management is not about reacting to the dominant paradigm or making fear based decisions. It is not about learning skills "in case daddy punishes us," or out of fear of "daddy forbidding us."

For me, fertility management is an ancestral legacy. It is a homesteading skill. It is a human right.

I have learned how to manage my fertility in order to co-create & participate in the world I want to live in motivated by love, not fear.

The Sacred Yes

Most people choose their method of contraception with a mindset rooted in fear, mis & disinformation. Most people choose their method of contraception rooted in the energy of "no."

No baby no baby no baby.

Our ability to say "no" to a conception or pregnancy is sacred, but fear based decision making can be toxic.

FUCK normalizing actions rooted in fear rather than love, especially when it comes to directing the power of our marvelous sexuality & fantastic fertility.

Healthy sexuality & fertility can connect us with immense pleasure & power.

This immense pleasure & power is innate to our biology.

To establish dynamic balance & wholeness we must move beyond the fearful "No" to identify & embrace the "Yes" that defines it as we avoid pregnancy.

"No" does not exist in a vacuum. **It is defined by what we actually want to say yes to.**

Our contraception practice & sexual experiences have the potential to be acts of ritual & mindfulness, invoking our Sacred Yes.

In order for our contraception & sexual experiences to invoke & embody our deepest intentions & desires we must identify, articulate, & honor our Sacred Yes.

By devoting our embodied actions to what we *do desire* instead of focusing what we *do not* want, we can shift our focus from fear to love. The same energetic capacity we have to feel sexual pleasure, orgasm, or create a child can be harnessed to achieve expansive states of consciousness & embodiment. It is possible to focus this energy to aid us in conceiving & birthing any number of creative, intellectual, spiritual, or practical pursuits.

Some folks call this "sex magic." Witchcraft, Tantra, Taoism, & Kabbalah are just a few of the traditions that have much to offer us for creating meaningful rituals for cultivating our sexual fertile power for healing & enlightenment.*

*see my Mapping The Yoniverse coloring book, Conscious Contraception Skillshare, or peruse the sacred sex & spirituality resources at the end of this work for further introduction to these traditions

Some questions to help you find your Sacred Yes:

✳   What helps you feel sexual power?

_____

_____

_____

_____

✳   What helps you feel abundant & fertile emotionally or spiritually?

_____

_____

_____

_____

✳   What is it that you want to spend your attention & energy engaged in besides being pregnant or parenting?

_____

_____

_____

✳ How do you most enjoy spending your time?

_____

_____

_____

✳ What activities bring you feelings of :
 • Joy
 • Aliveness
 • Connection
 • Fulfillment

_____

_____

_____

_____

✳ What do you desire to conceive, gestate, & birth that is not a child?

_____

_____

✳ Why do you want:
 • Intimacy
 • Orgasms
 • Penetration from somebody who creates sperm

_____

_____

_____

_____

* What do you value most about sexual experiences?

_____

_____

_____

_____

_____

* What do you want to experience more of in your life that would be impossible or difficult during pregnancy or parenting?

_____

_____

_____

_____

_____

Your answers to these questions will likely shift as your mood, lifestyle, partner(s), fertility cycle, & any other number of factors change. It's important to ask these questions consistently & without judging your authentic answers.

I recommend taking a moment to identify a Sacred Yes every single time you engage with sexual energy in your body.

This can be done silently within your mind & heart for a brief moment, spoken aloud, written on a sticky note aptly placed on a mirror, steering wheel, fridge or phone. Your Sacred Yes can be meditated on daily, & invoked while gathering data for your fertility awareness practice, or while in orgasmic states. A new level of intimacy can be reached when you exchange a Sacred Yes verbally with your partner on a regular basis, particularly before making love. You & your partner don't have to have the same Yes as long as you respect & appreciate each others'.

Ideally, I recommend clearly stating your Sacred Yes to your Self, Partner, & Spirit *before* each sexual experience, or as the sexual energy is beginning to rise. Stating this intention (along with where the sperm should go if any is to be ejaculated!) before sex is a powerful way to align your action with your intention.

Yes, Please Bleed!

If you do accidentally get sperm in your vagina during a potentially fertile time, you can engage with plants & practical magic to induce menstruation rooted in your Sacred Yes. Instead of moving from a place of fear of pregnancy (or fear of abortion), it is possible to engage with plants & practical magic with a loving, nourishing intention to maintain the integrity of the completely natural, normal process that is menstrual bleeding.

Yes to bleeding.

Yes to ovulating again in your next cycle.

Yes to body sovereignty.

Yes to all the things you want to conceive, gestate, & birth that are not a child.

Yes to shameless sexual pleasure & power.

Yes, Please Bleed!

"Caring for myself is not self-indulgence, it is self-preservation, & that is an act of political warfare."

Audre Lorde

Cultivating Consciousness: Birth Control vs. Contraception

I spent more than a decade of my life on-call for birth as a doula. My goal as a birth keeper was to support & facilitate a natural physiologic process, a feat which in the medical paradigm requires ninja skills of agile advocacy & deft defense. The modern medical paradigm controls birth with fearful, harmful power dynamics, narcotics, synthetic hormones, & surgery.

> **I abhor the words "birth" & "control" next to one another & would love to decrease their paired use in our language. Birth does not need to be controlled, it needs to be rewilded & reclaimed.**

Preventing ovulation is not controlling birth.

Instead of birth control, I use the term **contraception** to describe what I teach & practice.

contra ~ Latin for "against," to counter

conception ~ Old French, the act of conceiving in the womb
Clinically speaking: when an ovum is fertilized & creates a zygote.

I avoid using the term "birth control" to describe contraception. While "birth control" is perhaps the most popular widely understood term used to describe objects, medications, & methods for avoiding pregnancy, I prefer to use more accurate & descriptive terms. For example, I call synthetic hormonal contraception methods exactly what they are: **ovulation prevention methods**.

Synthetic hormonal contraception methods like the pill, patch, shot, or hormonal IUDs **do not control birth**, they destroy important endocrine function in order to **prevent ovulation**. Diminishing endocrine function & preventing ovulation has a myriad of adverse affects on our health, from microbiome & mineral absorption to bone density & mood, to the shrinking of our clitorus & ovaries.

All types of contraception, including synthetic hormones, have a purpose, time, & place when used with true informed consent. The medical system is an industry, not a healing modality. Most of us have not been taught to be conscious consumers from the medical industry. This is not the fault of individual consumers, it's a result of systemic oppression meant to keep us subjugated below false external authority.

> **"Do the best you can until you know better. When you know better, do better."**
>
> **Maya Angelou**

Plants as Allies for Promoting Menstruation, NOT as Contraception

Keeping sperm out of the vagina during the fertile phase is the best method I know of for preventing pregnancy. Full stop. Contrary to what popular belief & mainstream narratives may be, we are capable of effectively avoiding pregnancy without the aid of any inanimate objects or foreign substances. We'll discuss this further in the physiology section of this work.

Plant medicine is incredibly powerful, & ingesting it can affect many aspects of our mind, bodies, & spirit. Plants are not always gentle or benign.

I do not recommend using plants as a regular method of contraception.

Using plants regularly to prevent conception means using plants to:

* Interrupt ovulation

* Interrupt progesterone that naturally occurs after ovulation (which does not prevent conception, but implantation of a fertilized egg)

* As spermicide, which will also disrupt the delicate pH & microbiome of vaginal ecology

---

These processes either disrupt our hormonal cycle or disrupt our vaginal microbiome. Our hormonal balance & vaginal ecology are both vital & nuanced eco-systems in our body that deserve our nourishment & support for optimal health, not destruction.

Perhaps when we had shorter lifespans (fewer cycles within a lifetime) & less exposure to toxic endocrine disruptors in our environment (plastics, pesticides, conventional meat & dairy, etc.), working with plants to interfere with our hormonal cycle could have been less harmful. In today's highly toxic & stressful world I do not recommend consuming any substance, be it plant based or synthetic, to interfere with healthy natural hormone function. There are enough pollutants & toxins in our environment for our organ systems to cope with as it is.

In today's world, I believe it is vital we nurture, not disrupt, our body ecology, its hormones, & microbiome whenever possible, rather than knowingly interfere with it.

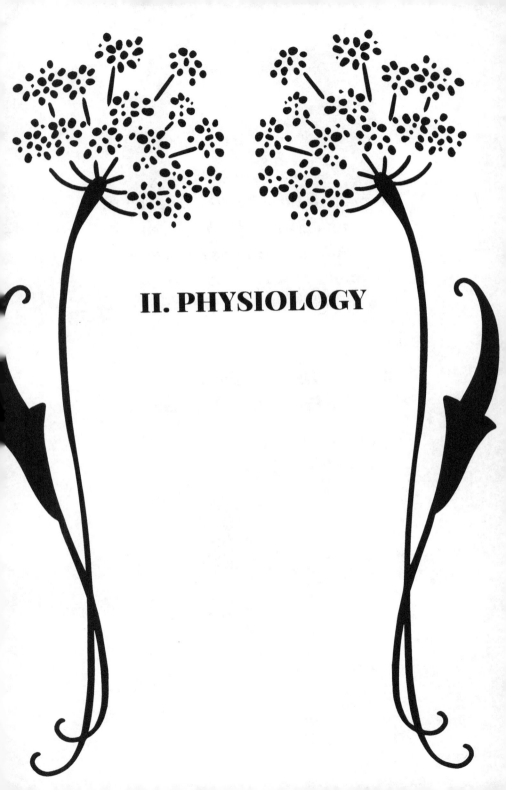

II. PHYSIOLOGY

"From a natural health perspective, my main criteria for birth control is that it not shut down ovulation. That it not shut down hormones. In other words, that it not castrate women."

Dr. Lara Briden
"The Period Revolutionary"

Fertility Awareness Method

The Sympto-thermal method of fertility awareness is a profoundly empowering option for contraception that has been found to be 99.4% effective when practiced correctly. I have been practicing this method for over 15 years at the time of writing this. I learned from a book at age 19 & never received any formal instruction. "Please Bleed!" is not meant to provide adequate instruction for safely practicing fertility awareness, but I wanted to include a brief summary of its basic tenets for anyone who might not be familiar with it.

The sympto-thermal method of fertility awareness tracks three biomarkers, also referred to as primary fertility signals:

*   **Cervical fluids.** Fertile fluids are the primary fertility signal; the most important bio-marker for identifying our fertile phase.

*   **Basal body temperature.** This spikes after we ovulate because of a surge in the hormone progesterone (more on this later). Our body temperature cannot predict ovulation or identify the fertile window, but it can confirm ovulation has occurred when taken consistently after at least 4 hours of sleep.

*   **Cervical position & texture.** This changes throughout the cycle. During the fertile window the cervix is softer & higher in the vagina than other times in the cycle.

By tracking these biomarkers one can detect both ovulation & the "fertile window." This "fertile window" is typically less than a week long, & varies from person to person, cycle to cycle. If one wishes to avoid pregnancy, one can abstain from sexual contact that allows sperm into the vagina during the fertile window. Ovulation itself happens in a moment, not over several days. After ovulation the egg is only alive for about a day, & that is the only time conception can take place. Occasionally (rarely) two or more eggs will pop within a 24 hour period, but never more than a day apart from one another. **If you have no contact with sperm during your fertile window you will not get pregnant.**

Voila.

For more detailed information please see my website to download a free e-book &/or print your free pdf of my "Ovulation Awareness" zine. You may also wish to join the Conscious Contraception Skillshare. I list some of my favorite wonderful fertility awareness instructors & texts for further study in the resource section.

Pleasure, Intimacy, & Contraception

Keeping sperm out of the vagina & off the vulva to avoid pregnancy does not mean practicing abstinence! As individuals & a collective, we need to let go of the penis-in-vagina-till-penis-ejaculates definition of sex. Sex & healthy sexuality are so much more than that.

Instead of abstaining from sexual activity entirely during the fertile phase of the cycle, I recommend employing a combination of creativity, critical thinking skills, & clear communication with both your self & sexual partner(s) to remain in alignment with one's intentions to avoid conception. Claiming & embodying your Sacred Yes is vital. Sexuality & pleasure during the fertile window present a unique opportunity to

enjoy exploring & playing with the infinite
intimate
erotic & orgasmic
activities that do not result in sperm on the vulva or in the vagina.

There are literally infinite ways we can celebrate, cultivate & explore sexual energy without danger of pregnancy. I dare you to start a personal list of erotic & pleasureable activities that do not risk pregnancy & could feel joyful for you!

Yum.

Oops!

If for whatever reason you are unable to keep sperm out of your vagina during the fertile window, you might conceive when you ovulate. That conception may become a pregnancy. **There is a distinct physiologic & energetic difference between a conception & a pregnancy.** You do not "get pregnant" when you conceive. Each conception has about an 80% chance of implanting successfully & becoming a pregnancy. That means that about 1 in 5 conceptions naturally pass without causing a pregnancy.

We are capable of tipping the odds in our favor if we'd rather bleed than gestate. We are capable of allying with emmenagogues & other holistic healing arts to help stimulate the release of our endometrium. While you would not know it, it's possible there could be a tiny zygote or blastocyst (fertilized egg) that may be floating around in the endometrium that has not yet implanted, & it could be released too.

The following section outlines the timeline & physiology of ovulation & conception. **Before attempting to interrupt the process of implantation with plants & practical magic, it is essential to understand the nuanced anatomy & physiology of our fertility, including ovulation, conception & implantation.**

Some zygotes will never make it down the egg tube at all, & will result in an ectopic pregnancy which can be a life threatening condition. Ectopic pregnancies can be detected with ultrasound.

The Fertile Window

* Approximately 6 days (maximum) prior to ovulation

* Fertile fluids are secreted from the cervix & become present in the vagina

* Cervix softens & rises in the vagina

Sperm can survive in fertile fluids for up to 6 days, therefore sperm entering the vagina when fertile fluids are present can result in conception, even when ovulation does not coincide with the sperm exposure.

Ovulation & Conception

* The egg is alive for about a day after the moment of ovulation.

* **Conception can only happen when the egg is alive.**

Progesterone & Body Temperature
(This is important)

* Whether or not conception takes place, the empty sac that once held the egg becomes an endocrine gland & begins to secrete **progesterone**.

* **Progesterone** raises the body's temperature to a level that helps support a fertilized egg's life in the womb. If one has been monitoring waking basal body temperature earlier in the cycle, this progesterone will create a visible spike in temperature the day of or after ovulation.

* Progesterone thickens the uterine lining.

* Pregnancy is not possible without adequate levels of progesterone.

* If there is no conception, the body temperature will go back down when progesterone levels fall just before menstruation begins.

* Progesterone levels must fall for menstruation to occur.

* If conception takes place, temperatures will remain higher than the usual baseline from the point of conception throughout pregnancy due to high levels of progesterone.

Pregnancy is not possible without adequate levels of progesterone.

The Golden Window

✱ It typically takes 3 days for the fertilized egg, at this stage scientifically called a *zygote*, to journey through the egg tube to the uterus.

✱ It takes another 6-10 days for the fertilized egg, at this stage scientifically called a *blastocyst*, to implant in the side of the uterine wall, & another 4 days to *securely* attach itself.

As discussed earlier, between 20-25% of all blastocysts never securely attach themselves to the uterine wall & pass in the following menstruation undetected without any adverse symptoms.

"The Golden Window" is not a technical or proper term, it's just one that I personally like to use to describe the special period of time after conception, before implantation. During this time the blastocyst has not connected to the maternal blood network or securely embedded itself in the endometrium. A large percentage of conceptions will naturally pass in the menstrual blood after this phase is complete, thus *working with plants & practical magic to tip the scale in your favor to bleed is not manipulating our physiology to do anything wildly out of the norm.*

Encouraging menstruation after a conception & prior to implantation will not usually present any signs of the conception such as clots, or fetal tissue. The fertilized ovum, called a *blastocyst*, will be undetectable in your menstrual flow.

Most pregnancy tests will not detect a pregnancy at this stage, so one must have been aware of their cycle, a potential conception, & take action promptly. **We cannot rely on external sources of authority or data at this stage, we must trust & follow our intuition & body awareness.**

THE GOLDEN WINDOW

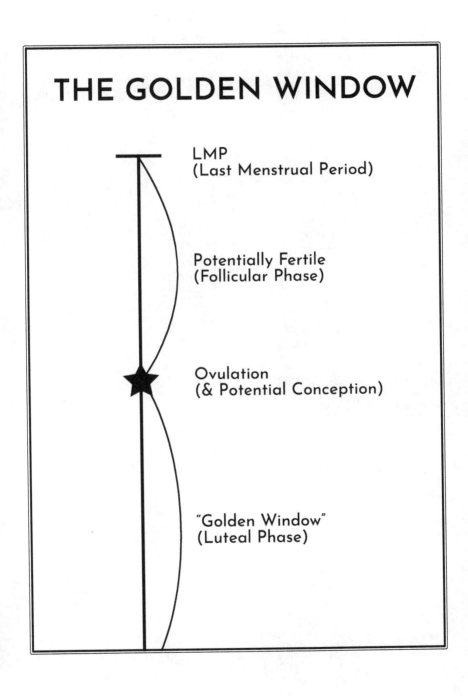

LMP
(Last Menstrual Period)

Potentially Fertile
(Follicular Phase)

Ovulation
(& Potential Conception)

"Golden Window"
(Luteal Phase)

The most common over-the-counter pharmaceutical emergency contraception pills, "Plan B," will not prevent implantation of an already fertilized egg during "the golden window." This is one reason why I prefer to work with plants & practical magic rather than pills during this stage. *It is worth noting that if you have not yet ovulated, the pills will usually prevent ovulation & thus conception from happening.*

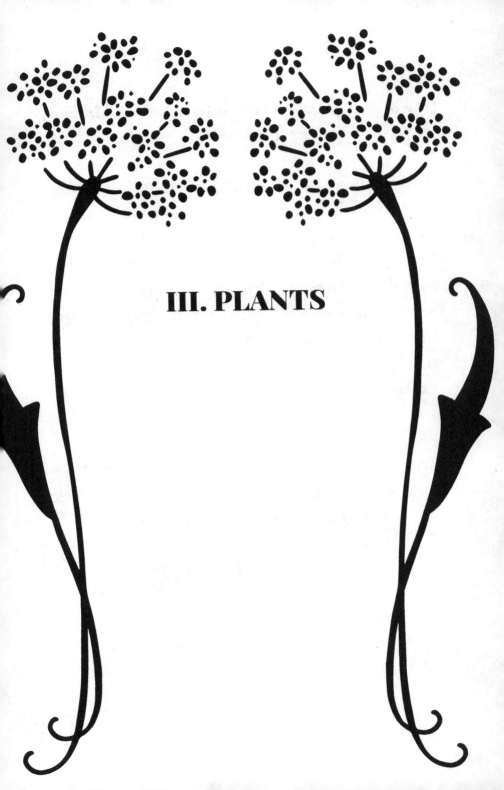

III. PLANTS

"One of our greatest fears is to eat the wildness of the world.

"Our mothers intuitively understood something essential: the green is poisonous to civilization. If we eat the wild, it begins to work inside us, altering us, changing us. Soon, if we eat too much, we will no longer fit the suit that has been made for us. Our hair will begin to grow long & ragged. Our gait & how we hold our body will change. A wild light begins to gleam in our eyes. Our words start to sound strange, nonlinear, emotional. Unpractical. Poetic.

"Once we have tasted this wildness, we begin to hunger for a food long denied us, & the more we eat of it the more we will awaken."

Stephen Buhner

Please Bleed!

Emmenagogue ~ Greek. *emména*, menses or month, *agógos*, drawing forth

The entire category of plants called "emmenagogues" are pro-menstruation, herbal options for saying "please bleed" to your body. The category of emmenagogue plants have a wide variety of properties & actions. Some emmenagogues are tonics, some affect hormonal activity, & others work through irritation & stimulation of uterine tissues. Most emmenagogues increase general blood flow throughout the body, or specifically in the pelvis.

Emmenagogues are excellent allies within a Conscious Contraception practice. Even in the case of an "oops," if we are working with plants to prevent implantation or a subsequent pregnancy, we can do so rooted in The Sacred Yes of cycle promotion rather than pregnancy destruction.

The Power of Plant Medicine

There is a common misconception that herbs are always gentle, or provide a more "natural" alternative way to do what pharmaceuticals do. This is not true. Many plants are incredibly powerful & will create dramatic effects. **Plants do not replace pills. Plants are people* too. They are sentient & have personalities.**

Herbs can be taken in many forms, including but not limited to tinctures made from alcohol or glycerin, tea infusions, vinegar tonics, or capsules. Herbal baths infused with strong tea are another delightful way to immerse yourself in plant medicine's healing power.

Plant medicine demands thoughtful & respectful use. If you are interested in going deeper with plant medicine it is ideal to create a personal, intimate, relationship with plants local to your specific bioregion, or perhaps even your ancestral lands.

Ideally, consult an experienced herbalist before beginning any intensive herbal regimen.

*I do not mean that plants have human qualities (anthropomorphism), rather, that plants have personhood (animism).

Honoring Our Elders & Embracing Our Allies

Plants are our elders. With intention, effort, & presence they can become our allies, teachers, & friends. The use of plant medicine, when approached with astute self awareness & respect for the sentience of the plants, has the potential to deepen human reverence for the intricate web of interconnected life.

By choosing to work with plants rather than pharmaceuticals, we have the opportunity to seek synergy with our natural environment rather than consume from an industry that actively destroys it. While the dominant paradigm of western medicine uses pills & surgeries to "cure" us of our fertility, plant medicine can be used to promote menstruation & the integrity of the natural womb cycle.

Plants, Embodiment & Intention

If you would like to work with plants to induce menstruation & avoid pregnancy, it is important to make a serious dedicated effort to align your physical & psycho-spiritual body. Whether this is through movement practices, prayer, meditation, or ritual, ensuring that your devotion & commitment to the process at hand is fortified fully by your will is vital.

You are not a passive participant in this process.

You must identify with the process & fully align with it.

Plants are not pills that you can simply "take" to complete a desired effect.

Plants are allies & elders that can assist us in our quest for embodied intention.

Desired Herbal Actions employed to "Please Bleed!" During The Golden Window:

✶ **Inhibit Progesterone.** As discussed earlier, *pregnancies are not possible without progesterone*. Without enough progesterone the uterine lining will not be thick, or the body warm, enough to sustain pregnancy.

✶ **Increase Estrogen.** This upsets hormonal balance & ratio between estrogen & progesterone, which ultimately serves to inhibit progesterone.

✶ **Stimulate & Move The Lining of the Uterus.** Increase blood flow to the pelvis by
  • relaxing or contracting the muscles of the uterus with oxytocin or increased circulation, or
  • agitating the mucosa of the endometrium

HERBAL ACTIONS

Throughout the upcoming materia medica section you will see the following symbols to indicate the following herbal actions:

Inhibit Progesterone

As discussed earlier, pregnancies are not possible without progesterone. Without enough progesterone the uterine lining will not be thick, or the body warm, enough to sustain pregnancy.

Increase Estrogen

This upsets hormonal balance & ratio between estrogen & progesterone, which ultimately serves to inhibit progesterone.

Stimulate & Move

Circulation: stimulate & move blood

Oxytocin: stimulate & move nerves & muscles

Irritation: stimulate & move mucosal tissue

Timing

To promote menstrual bleeding in the case of an "Oops!," my practice has been to begin a dedicated regimen with strong emmenagogues from each of the 3 categories mentioned above at the start of a normal cycle's 4th week, or around 21 days after your last menstrual cycle. During this week of the cycle the body remembers a dramatic hormonal shift, & working with plants can encourage that shift to happen.

Queen Anne's Lace or Rue, discussed in the following pages, may be taken immediately after ovulation for anywhere from a few days to a full week to inhibit progesterone & therefore implantation. However, if I were very serious about desiring menstruation rather than an embryo formation or implantation after I suspected conception, I would personally work with stronger emmenagogues consistently in the 4th week of the cycle, about one week after ovulation & one week before my period was due, until bleeding began.

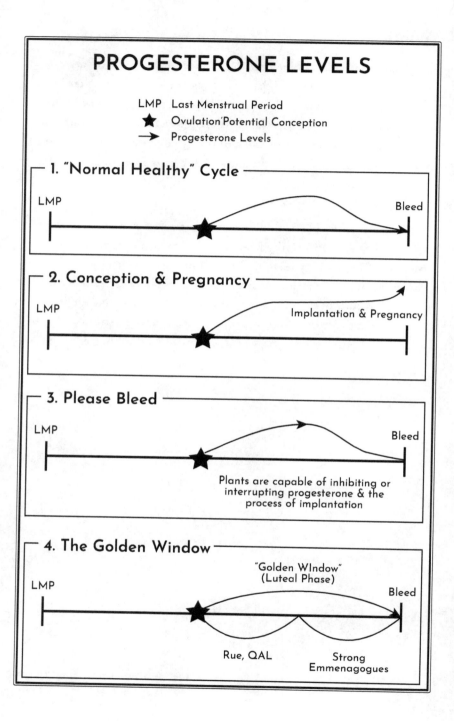

PROGESTERONE LEVELS

LMP — Last Menstrual Period
★ — Ovulation/Potential Conception
→ — Progesterone Levels

1. "Normal Healthy" Cycle

LMP

Bleed

2. Conception & Pregnancy

LMP

Implantation & Pregnancy

3. Please Bleed

LMP

Bleed

Plants are capable of inhibiting or
interrupting progesterone & the
process of implantation

4. The Golden Window

LMP

"Golden WIndow"
(Luteal Phase)

Bleed

Rue, QAL

Strong
Emmenagogues

Formulas & Dosage

For plant medicines to be effective they must be taken consistently. Most regimens involve dosing every 3 to 4 hours for anywhere from a few days to a week to achieve the desired effect upon your body's chemistry & tissues. This usually looks like dosing 3 to 5 times per day. Some plants prefer to be ingested with food, & some without. Some folks like to wake up in the night to take doses consistently, but I do not recommend this as the value of deep sleep in nourishing our full beings cannot be overstated.

I do not recommend specific formulas or dosage in this work for good reason. There is no "one size fits all" formula or regimen for our endeavor of promoting menstrual bleeding. Furthermore, I do not know your constitution, which plants grow in your region, or which plants are traditionally used in your lineage. Please explore these things & seek out an experienced herbalist to help you create an appropriate formula & regimen unique to you.

There are literally hundreds if not thousands of plants that might help us bring on menstruation in case of an "oops." I outline a dozen or so of my own closest allies in the following pages. Most of them are somewhat easy to access, whether via retail online, in herb or natural food stores, or growing in your own neighborhood. I suggest choosing a plant that fulfills the action of each of the 3 categories discussed above to build your formula or regimen.

I like to work with gentle, small doses of these plants cyclically whether or not I have had an "Oops" to help my body acquaint them with bleeding. For example, I'll take a dropper full of Angelica tincture 3x daily for a few days leading up to my normal menstrual bleeding to help encourage & support its flow.

Care & Caution

Before using herbal allies to avoid or disrupt implantation I advise the following precautions & protocols:

* Consult & work with an experienced herbalist before trying any new herbal regimen.

* Understand the contraindications & signs of toxicity associated with your choice of plants.

* Have a caring companion accessible not just by telephone, but physically present to support your well-being. Someone committed to checking in on you multiple times a day, as often as every few hours.

* Work with an herbalist who is well versed in constitutional assessment, and potentially have muscle testing to discern which remedies are best for you

* Be aware of the risk of an incomplete process & sketch out a plan of action. Explore options for addressing a subsequent pregnancy. Have a back-up plan appointment with your womb wellness care provider of choice.

* Be aware of how much blood is too much blood to be losing (generally this is more than 2 overnight pads per hour) & have a plan of action to address excessive blood loss.

* Drink lots of water!

* Have a kidney & liver rehab plan ready to nourish & cleanse these organ systems which are heavily taxed by hormonal loads & most strong emmenagogues. Food as medicine, plant allies, & Chinese medicine are particularly adept.

General Signs of Toxicity

✳ Because many emmenagogues are muscle relaxants, some loose stool is to be expected. However, diarrhea that's prolonged for more than three days can be a serious issue leading to dehydration.

✳ Other signs of toxicity include prolonged symptoms such as: dull frontal headache (especially with black cohosh), excessive nausea (many of these plants aggravate morning sickness), abdominal cramping (in the gut, not the pelvis), fever or temperature fluctuation, decreased or increased heart rate.

✳ See protocols above, & know that hyper awareness of your own body & an objective observer are essential!

Materia Medica

Implantation Inhibitors

Queen Anne's Lace & Rue are considered implantation inhibitors most effective *directly after ovulation*, when progesterone levels naturally spike with or without conception. It is vital to understand the distinction that these plants potentially prevent implantation, not conception.

Queen Anne's Lace *Daucus carota*

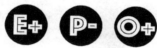

Queen Anne's Lace works to inhibit implantation because it is estrogenic, oxytocic, & inhibits progesterone production. Progesterone is one of, if not, *the* most important hormone needed to sustain pregnancy. Queen Anne's Lace has been used for over 2000 years as an implantation inhibitor in India & the Appalachian mountains. The oldest reference of its use as contraception is from Hippocrates. Chewing the seeds is reportedly more effective for preventing implantation & pregnancy than tea or tincture preparations. Grinding with a mortar & pestle or electric device to crush the seeds would also work to release the special aromatic terpenes. This method of implantation inhibition works best for people with regular menstrual cycles.

Plant parts used for implantation inhibition: Seeds (sometimes accompanied by flowers, but main constituents are in the seed)

Clinical Actions

* Aromatic

* Carminative (affects digestive tract)

* Diuretic - makes you pee!

* Urinary antiseptic (helpful for healing UTIs)

Energetics: very dry & warming

Tissues: gut, reproductive, & endocrine

Contraindications

* Volatile oils can irritate the kidneys/bladder over long periods of time

* Excessively drying to already-dry constitutions

* Can affect progesterone levels

* Dehydration, constipation

For more extensive information about Queen Anne's Lace (QAL) see the resource section; Robin Rose Bennet's work, & QAL zine & online class by my dear friend & teacher Ms. Molly Dutton Kenny.

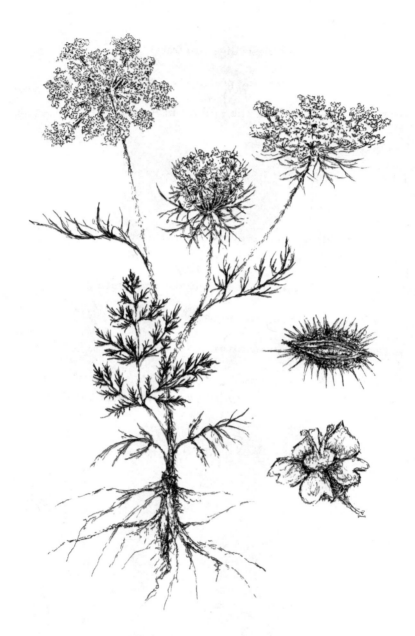

Daucus carota

Rue *Ruta graveolens*

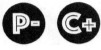

Rue's name is derived from the Greek *reuo*, meaning 'to set free.'

Rue contains Rutin, which stimulates adrenaline, hardens bones & teeth, & strengthens arteries & veins. This hardening effect, in combination with increased adrenaline, decreases capillary capacity around the uterus & inhibits blood flow & nourishment to the lining, & therefore is effective as an implantation inhibitor.

In Western traditions, this plant has long been associated with the Roman goddess Diana who is sometimes called the "Queen of Witches." Diana is a Triple Goddess: Virgin Moon, Mother of all Creatures, & Crone Destroyer. In diverse cultures the world over, Rue has lore as both a love charm, abortifacient, & amulet against evil spirits.

Plant parts used for emmenagogue & implantation inhibition: leaves & new shoots

Clinical Actions & Indications

* ✶ Uterine stimulant for damp qi stagnation

* ✶ Amenorrhea, a fancy word for not bleeding

* ✶ Spasmodic dysmenorrhea, a fancy word for irregular or painful bleeding

* ✶ Antiparasitic

Energetics: dry, aromatic & stimulating

Tissues: uterus, liver, kidney, GI

Contraindications

* Can cause photosensitivity/ rashes with exposure to sunlight

* Should not be used even clinically for more than 2 weeks because of extreme risk of toxicity

* Potential to cause vomiting, do not take after eating

* Anyone with liver, heart, or kidney troubles **should not** use this herb

* Multiple deaths via organ system failure associated with overdose

* May increase anxiety & fear from stimulated levels of adrenaline & fight or flight response which can be taxing to the adrenals

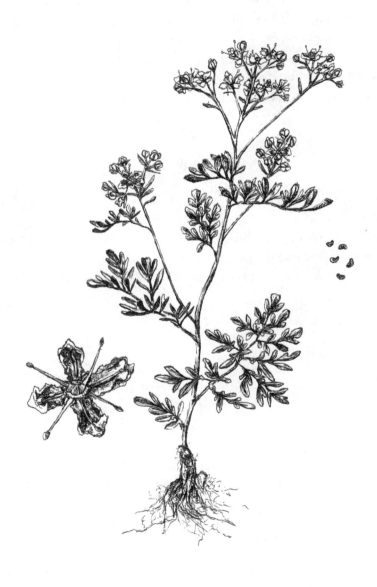

Ruta graveolens

Thujone

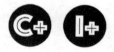

A volatile oil found in several plants & known to be a uterine stimulant. Anyone with a tendency toward epileptic seizures **should not**
use herbs containing thujone. Mugwort*, wormwood, tansy, juniper,
& red cedar are just a few examples of plants that contain Thujone.

*There are enough volatile oils in the plants themselves, do not use essential oils of any
of these plants internally.*

Clinical Actions

* Emmenagogic/abortifacient, probably via irritation of mucosa

* Uterine contractor

* These plants can be effective when used as a hot infusion
  for several days prior to anticipated period, especially with
  ginger

Energetics: tend to be dry

Tissues: various, though all aromatics affect the mucous membranes
as counter-irritants

Contraindications

* ✴ Hard on the liver

* ✴ Irritates the kidneys

* ✴ Large doses are psychoactive

* ✴ Contraindicated for excessively hot/dry constitutions

* ✴ Tansy (a perennial plant) specifically associated with: nausea vomiting, inflamed stomach lining, phototoxic (sensitive to sunlight)

*Mugwort, Artemisia vulgaris came to me in a dream before the final edits of this book & asked to be given greater acknowledgement in this work. This bitter warming plant has been used throughout the ages in ceremony & ritual to court the veil, for dreamwork, & womb care. Associated with the goddess Artemis, moon goddess of the hunt & protector of women in pregnancy & birth. The leaves or flowers of this plant can be imbibed as a tincture or tea, or applied as smoke medicine called moxabustion, as discussed in the "practical magic" section. Mugwort is a powerful emmenagogue, stimulating, tonifying, & bringing heat & energy to the womb.

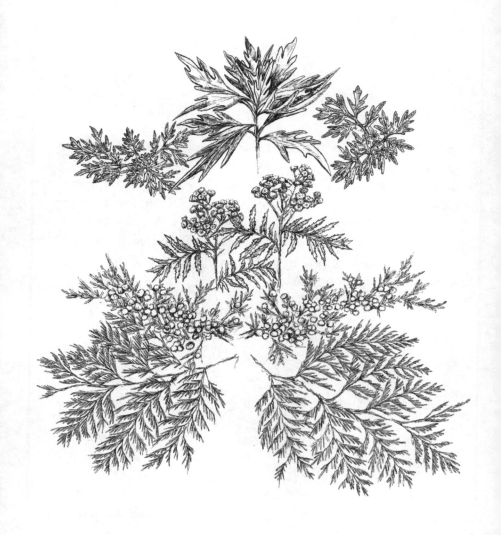

Thujone

Angelica *Angelica sinensis*

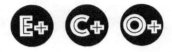

Also called "bellyache root," Don Quai, or dead nettle. Angelica has also been called "the root of holy ghost," & sometimes called "the female ginseng." She is a member of the parsley family, so likely very high in vitamin C also, which is said to help inhibit progesterone. This plant can increase menstrual bleeding & should be used with caution or not at all by anyone who already experiences heavy bleeding with their cycle.

Plant parts used for emmenagogue: roots & seeds

Clinical Actions

*   Stimulates circulation

*   Estrogenic & oxytocic

*   Can relax or contract smooth muscles depending on preparation. Prepared as a hot water infusion it is a stimulant which is ideal for trying to post an eviction notice.

Energetics: warm, stimulating, dry, very moving

Tissues: smooth muscles

Contraindications & Signs of Toxicity

* Blood clots

* Liver toxicity

* Dilation of pupils

* Stomach ache

* Excessive menstrual bleeding

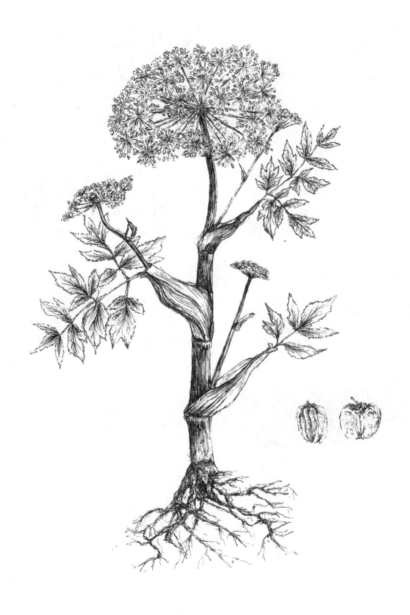

Angelica sinensis

Pennyroyal *Mentha pulegium*

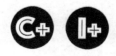

A lovely tummy soother in the mint family with a deadly reputation due to uneducated desperate individuals attempting to induce abortion by taking the essential oil internally, which can cause kidney failure. It's been used & known as an emmenagogue & abortifacient for centuries, made famous in our contemporary age by the 90s Nirvana song "Pennyroyal Tea." It can be used as an emmenagogue by making a strong tea to drink &/or adding to bathwater. DO NOT TAKE ESSENTIAL OIL INTERNALLY. Essential oil may be used externally for belly massage within a carrier oil, under a castor oil pack, or added to bath water.

Parts used as emmenagogue: leaves & flower tops

Clinical Actions

* Stimulating emmenagogue for amenorrhea & spasmodic dysmenorrhea

* Relaxing stimulant

* Especially effective when used in tandem with one of the Thujone containing plants

Energetics: very aromatic, dry

Tissues: GI, reproductive

Contraindications

* As an essential oil contains the ketone pulegone which is neurotoxic as well as toxic to the liver & kidneys in large amounts

* Very hard on the kidneys, liver & nervous system

* Do not take for more than 5 days

* Nausea is a common side effect

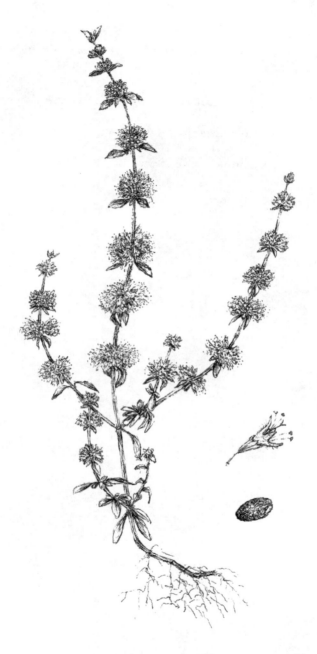

Mentha pulegium

Black Cohosh *Cimicifuga racemosa*

Also known as Black Snake Root, this is known as an underworld plant. She helps with journeying to or surfacing from darkness, confronting our fears, demons, & negative beliefs: which must be witnessed & understood before they can be overcome!

Parts used for emmenagogue: roots

Clinical Actions

* Antispasmodic

* Nervine

* Antidepressant for types of hormone-related depression

* Relaxes the smooth muscles (which the uterus is made of)

* Estrogenic

Energetics: slightly warm & dry, relaxant

Tissues: muscles & nerves, endocrine system, specifically used for softening the cervix

Contraindications & Signs of Toxicity

* Trusted sources have warned me that this is a low dose plant, even when used clinically, as in no more than 10 drops of the tincture per dose

* Severe mood shifts

* Abdominal pain

* Blood clotting

* You know you've taken too much if you get a dull frontal headache

*Black + blue cohosh are traditionally used together to stimulate labor at full term, & may have an affinity for one another in formulas.

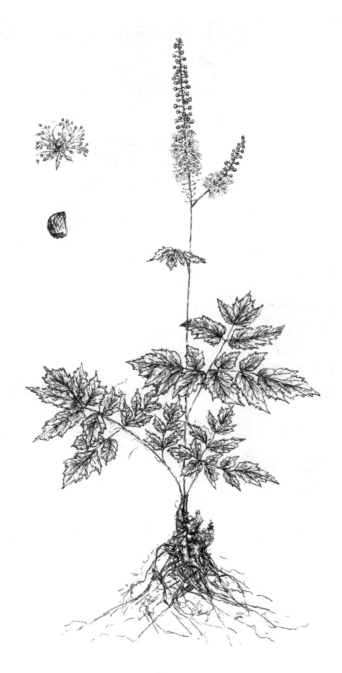

Cimicifuga racemosa

Blue Cohosh *Caulophyllum thalictroides*

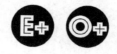

Because of its association with Native American women & their management of all types of womb care, historically this plant has been called papoose root. It is safely & commonly used to stimulate & expedite labor for pregnant women who are at term. Native Americans & Amish are both known to begin drinking this regularly about 2 weeks before their estimated due date. Blue cohosh is also used in formulas to treat endometriosis, chlamydia & cervical dysplasia. I usually combine it with red raspberry leaf for my birth clients at term.

Parts used as emmenagogue: root

Clinical action

* Estrogenic

* Oxytocic

* Regulation of menstrual cycle & easing of painful cramps

* Uterine tonic & stimulant

Energetics: warm & dry, stimulating, relaxing

Tissues: muscles & nerves; uterine stimulant encouraging contractions

Contraindications & Signs of Toxicity

* ✳ Problematic when taken with conventional birth control pills

* ✳ Narrows the arteries to the heart & **should not** be used with blood pressure issues or history of heart attack. Tends to lower blood pressure

* ✳ Headaches

* ✳ Nausea

* ✳ Dilated pupils

* ✳ Cardiovascular collapse

* ✳ Sore throat

* ✳ Muscle weakness

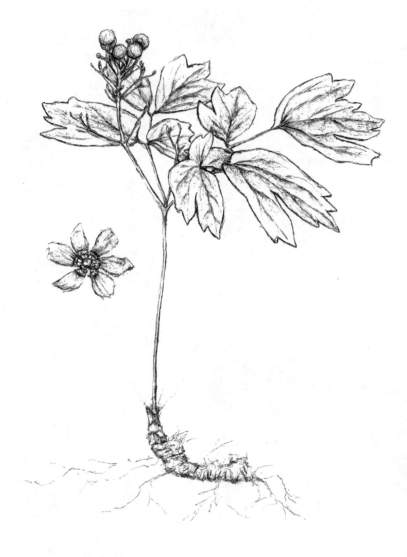

Caulophyllum thalictroides

Cotton root bark
Gossypium herbaceum

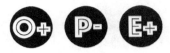

South American Creoles, Alabama Native Americans, & enslaved Africans on cotton plantations have used this as a contraceptive. It's very hard to find over the counter today but can be ordered online, or prepared at home if you have a good organic source.

Parts used for emmenagogue: root

Clinical Actions

* Astringent, very acidic

* Strong stimulant of uterine contraction/oxytocic

* Estrogenic + inhibits progesterone

* Believed to have fewer negative side effects on other organ systems than other common strong emmenagogues

Energetics: warm & dry

Tissues: endocrine, muscular skeletal system

Contraindications & Signs of Toxicity

* The book *Natural Liberty* says it has been proven to show atrophy of uterine tissue with repeated use

* Contains a chemical called gossypol which is toxic, but is counteracted by bioavailable iron: therefore, if taken (in addition to any abortifacients & blood flow promoting herbs!!) increase bioavailable iron intake as well

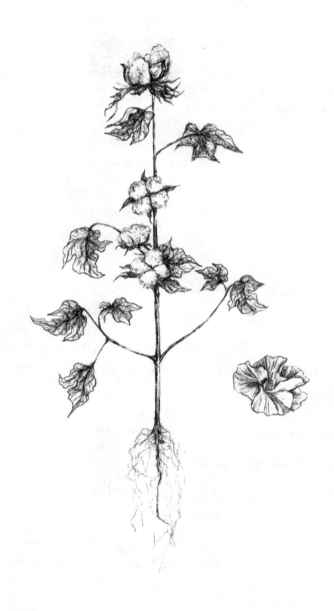

Gossypium herbaceum

Support Staff & Honorable Mention

Motherwort *Leonurus cardiaca*

The leaves & flowers of this plant are a bitter nervine. They can help with anxiety & all aspects of emotional & energetic "mothering" — an energy we need to turn inward to nurture ourselves. It's a relaxing stimulant for the uterus, the kidneys, & digestion, which soothes the physical & emotional heart.

Raspberry Leaf *Rubus idaeus or strigosus*

The leaves of the raspberry plant are a gentle tonic that nourish the uterine muscles & lining. They are also high in minerals. This plant can be used safely throughout the menstrual cycle, before, during, & after bleeding.

Yarrow *Achillea millefolium*

Moderates, slows, or instigates bleeding as needed. She helps hold energetic boundaries. Yarrow tones the reproductive system, heals tissue & prevents excess bleeding.

Red Cedar *Thuja plicata*

Often referred to as "Grandmother Cedar" in folk & indiginous traditions. She is centering & grounding. Cedar leaves contain Thujone & there are ethnobotanical reports of a concentrated decoction being used as an emmenagogue among Indigenous people.

Cascara Sagrada *Rhamnus purshiana*

This plant promotes a powerful downward motion, is a laxative, helps us release stuck emotions & energies, & promotes relaxation. Empirically, many women have reported menstruating early simply after meditating with this plant.

Red Cedar & Cascara Sagrada work really well in combination. Both of them LOVE to take the things that are not serving us, whether physical or emotional, & transform them.

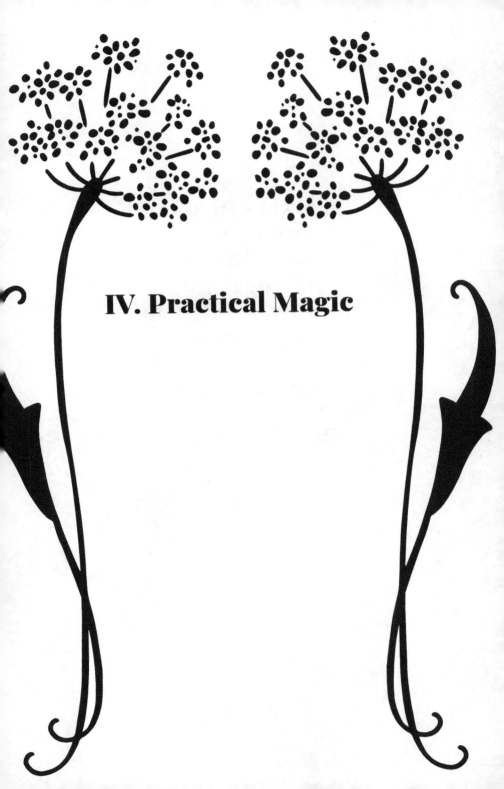

IV. Practical Magic

"All that you touch
You Change.
All that you Change
Changes you.
The only lasting truth
is Change.
God
is Change."

Octavia E. Butler

The art of magic has diverse definitions & practices, but almost always includes the use of ritual action for the purpose of shifting realities in the material plane to align with our individual intentions or will. The following suggestions include both practical scientifically proven methods for encouraging the opening & emptying of the womb, along with some more esoteric creative ideas for ritual.

* Root all your actions in your Sacred Yes; consider creating a mantra from one or more of your Sacred Yeses, or simply lovingly repeating the mantra "Please Bleed!"

* Stay warm & active. Excellent circulation is key to moving blood/qi. Wear extra layers, taking care especially to keep your low belly, low & mid-back cozy. All your organs in those areas need support via circulation to do their work. Staying warm is essential for your body's natural healing abilities to flourish. Dress warmly.

* Direct application of heat improves circulation & is highly effective for pain relief as well. Place one of the following on your lower belly or back:
  · Hot water bottle
  · Rice or buckwheat pillow warmed in the microwave
  · Electric heating pad
  · Warm Stones

* Use approximately 1-3 drops of essential oil to a large tablespoon of carrier oil, blend, & massage deeply into the flesh of the belly to help move blood & energy. Pennyroyal, Clary Sage, Red Cedar, & any of the Thujone family are appropriate for this application along with many other more soothing options like chamomile, lavender, or rose. (see pg 52 for more information about Thujone)

* Massage essential oil as described above in a carrier oil before heat application via stones, hot water bottle, etc.

* Enjoy spicy warming foods such as ginger & cayenne, hot soups & teas.

* Exercise vigorously.

* Receive reiki &/or other energy work

* Take hot baths infused with your herbal allies.

* Vaginal Steaming, especially with Thujone containing plants (fresh or dried herbs only, *do not steam with essential oils!*)

* Receive bodywork or treatments from Chinese & Asian healing modalities that employ our energy meridians, including but not limited to acupuncture or shiatsu, moxibustion, & Thai massage.

* Work with Chinese medicine energy meridians by applying direct pressure, circular massage, acupressure seeds (radish is commonly used), acupressure tacs, or moxibustion (smoke from dried & specially prepared mugwort) to acupressure points to promote bleeding; including but not limited to Spleen 6 & Large Intestine 4. See *Woman Heal Thyself* for more details, or research "the forbidden points" if you don't have a care-provider to offer instruction. Acupuncture needling is splendid also, though other methods mentioned here can be done independently with little to no financial investment.

* Work with flower essences for psycho-spiritual & energetic support. Love Lies Bleeding & Gentian are two possibilities to consider, but your needs will be unique.

* Orgasms! The best! Improves circulation, boosts mood & immune function, contracts the uterus.

* Meditation, Journaling, Reflection, Prayer

* Ritual

* Create an altar in your home focused on your intention to "Please Bleed!" This can be as simple or complex as you'd like. Sit in front of this altar & meditate or journal about your "Sacred Yes" daily. Create a collage from natural items, or magazines, represent pertinent deities you have or want to cultivate relationship with, honor your plant allies, & the elements.

Simple DIY Ritual Outline

Inspired by Reclaiming Witchcraft, European, & Native American traditions.

* **Plan & Clarify Intention**
  - **Who:** Humans to be present, &/or deity/spirits to be invoked
  - **What:** Objects, elements, colors, symbols
  - **Where:** What space & location?
  - **Why:** Create a clear statement of intention

* **Create sacred space & open the ritual**
  - Burning incense &/or clearing plants (ex: cedar, palo santo, sage, suggested to use local plants &/or plants specific to your lineage)
  - Calling the directions
  - Casting a circle (salt, smoke, candles, flowers, or simply visualization)
  - Offer prayers / words & intention to the divine
  - Invoke Deities or the divine to aid you
  - Making an altar space/including physical items or symbols of importance to you. Some like to represent all the elements, or include an image of a deity figure. Can be as simple or elaborate as you like.

* **Grounding – use a meditation, breathwork, &/or physical action to:**
  - Connect with the earth
  - Become fully present in your breath & body

* **Action ~ this can be anything meaningful for you! The following are just a few suggestions**
  - Song
  - Yoga, Dance, or other movement practices
  - Special Meditation or Prayer work

* **Using the elements to move energy symbolically**
  - Water ~ bathing your body, infusing herbs for tea, casting an object into moving water
  - Fire ~ burning objects, lighting a ritual hearth or candles
  - Earth ~ burying or planting something
  - Air ~ breath work, song
* **Closing of the Ritual / Opening of Circle**
  - Release & thank any energies invoked
  - Cleanse self & or circle with same or different action as opening

"Any ritual is an opportunity for transformation.

To do a ritual, you must be willing to be transformed in some way. The inner willingness is what makes the ritual come alive & have power.

If you aren't willing to be changed by the ritual, don't do it."

Starhawk

After Care Considerations

The aftercare considerations should actually be considered through-out the entire process & implemented as able:

*   Support your organ systems by eating only simple nutrient dense whole foods. Place emphasis on eating mineral rich items to replenish blood. Root veggies, bone broths, & dark leafy greens are a good place to start. Avoid all refined food products such as white flours, sugar, or anything that comes in a plastic package or out of a fryer

*   Stay hydrated! Adding a bit of salt, trace minerals, or hibiscus to your water can help with this

*   Consider working with plant medicines like dandelion, milk thistle, & burdock to help cleanse organ systems that may have had a higher than normal load of hormones to process

*   Red raspberry leaf is one wonderful plant that may be freely taken throughout our cycles to support uterine health

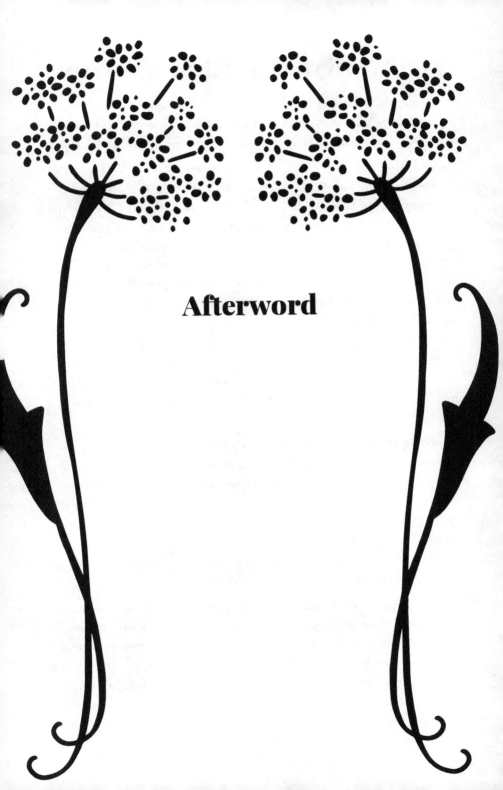

Afterword

Demystifying Herbal Abortion

Learning the details of materia medica, physiology, biochemistry, & energetics of implantation inhibition ought to give one a foundational understanding of how herbal abortion practices can work.

While this offering is not meant to provide *instruction* for how to create an herbal abortion, "Please Bleed!" does in fact offer the precise *information* needed to understand the *mechanisms* of how herbal abortions *can* work; by altering the body's hormonal baseline, stimulating circulation, stimulating uterine contractions, &/or irritating mucosa (endometrium) to expel it. The biochemical actions of plant medicine are not discerning between endometrium that would be released with normal menstruation & endometrium with the presence of a floating blastocyst or even an embedded embryo. Thujone will irritate mucosa. Estrogenic plants will inhibit progesterone (remember this as a 'pro-gestation' hormone), oxytocic plants will increase the potential of coordinated uterine contractions. As stated earlier, many emmenagogues may be used as abortifacients by altering the dosage & timing.

Posting an eviction notice in the uterus *after* implantation has occurred (a menstrual period has been missed) is often more toxifying, painful, time consuming, & less frequently effective at completely emptying the womb. An incomplete herbal abortion with retained tissue presents a myriad of risks including but not limited to infection, hemorrhage, organ failure (mainly due to toxicity carried by liver & kidneys), & most significantly : still being pregnant when you do not wish to be.

It is my educated opinion that using plant medicine to abort a pregnancy after implantation has occurred is not a wise choice for most individuals, especially those who have no previous intimate relationship with plant medicine. Objectively speaking, plant medicine is simply not the most effective vehicle for taking a direct route from point A (pregnant) to point B (not pregnant) available to us in modern times.

A dear & trusted teacher of mine has seen attempts at herbal abortion after implantation has occured to be about 40% effective in her practice. Even when successful, the process usually takes between 2 to 3 weeks of consistent dosing, & frequently includes significant physical & psycho-spiritual fatigue.

In contrast to those dismal success rates for complete herbal abortion after implantation, it is my personal (not professional!) experience that consistent intelligent dosing with herbs prior to a missed period has been 100% effective at bringing on menstruation after sperm exposure. Of course, I & the friends I've supported had no evidence that we had conceived. We were relying on our self awareness (knowledge of our fertile window, ovulation, & estimated due date for our next menses), intuition, & internal authority.

I am not a lawyer & I do not give legal advice, but it is my understanding that without a positive pregnancy test, i.e. what could be deemed "a clinically diagnosable pregnancy"* in a court of law, working with plants to stimulate menstruation is legal. It is a home remedy for bringing on menstruation, not an abortion. This distinction is important because the legal consequences of using herbs after implantation to terminate a pregnancy that has been confirmed can be severe. In some states herbal abortions can be considered felonies, practicing medicine without a licence, or homicide. Research your local laws, & contact If When How, an organization devoted to the legal defense of self induced abortion, for more information.

If we don't know our options, we don't have any. Herbal abortion is an option, & we ought not pretend otherwise. Being able to discern the true risks & benefits of our options wisely is contingent upon being provided with adequate education & support.

*This term "diagnosable pregnancy" is an official legal one. It speaks volumes of the oppressive pathologizing of our fertility prevalent in the dominant culture. Insurance industries quite literally regard pregnancy as a disease, or "pre-existing condition." Even when we are avoiding pregnancy, it is not a disease that needs to be treated with pills & surgery, it is a natural function of a healthy, fertile, sexual body.

Author's Note

Beyond the desire to provide accurate information, I have written "Please Bleed!" motivated by a longing to share the epic *feelings* I have gained from many years of engaging with a contraception practice that relies completely on self awareness, clear communication with a loving partner, & plants as Plan B.

I feel so fucking free.

I feel viscerally unafraid of pregnancy.

I feel sexually liberated & satisfied.

I feel deliciously politically subversive.

I feel intimately connected with my own body & being.

I feel aligned with & aware of the divine creative energy that animates all things.

I feel joyful & capable.

I feel rooted in my Sacred Yes.

I don't want to place my feelings on a pedestal or make them your aspirational goal. I just want to share with you that it is *possible* to feel this way about your contraception.

How do you want to feel?

What are the small immediately actionable steps you can take right now to make your life & contraception practice conducive to your desired feelings?

You deserve education, respect, & infinite kindness for your process, however it unfolds.

Your path to claiming the pleasure & power innate to your fertile sexual body will be as unique as your Sacred Yes. The risks &

benefits of your fertility management choices, like all life & health choices, are completely individual & nuanced.

It's an honor to share some of the wisdom & knowledge I have gathered in "Please Bleed!" I do so humbly with ownership of the fact that my personal truths are not universal. It is my greatest wish that my work will inspire you on your path to discovering your own personal truths, as well as cultivate the knowledge, skills, & support required to embody them.

In service to our healing & liberation,

Sam

"What value & respect do we give to our bodies? What uses do we have for them? What relation do we see, if any, between body & mind, or body & soul? What connections or responsibilities do we maintain between our bodies & the earth? These are religious questions, obviously, for our bodies are part of the Creation, & they involve us in all the issues of mystery. But the questions are also agricultural, for no matter how urban our life, our bodies live by farming; we come from the earth & return to it, & so we live in agriculture as we live in flesh. While we live our bodies are moving particles of the earth, joined inextricably both to the soil & to the bodies of other living creatures."

Wendell Berry

Glossary of Terms

Ovulation

The moment that the ovum, or egg, emerges from the ovary.

Endocrine

A system of glands that secrete hormones, located throughout the body.

Microbiome

From Greek terms meaning "tiny life." This term is used to refer to the existence & activity of microorganisms such as bacteria & viruses in our bodies.

Endometrium

The inner most layer of the uterus which is made of mucousy tissue & grows & sloughs in response to the hormonal cycle. Endometrium is released with healthy normal menstruation, & is held to nourish a growing pregnancy.

Implantation

In this work, this term refers to the process of the fertilized egg or blastocyst connecting itself securely to the wall of the uterus & maternal blood network.

Conception

The moment that a sperm fertilizes an egg.

Progesterone

An important hormone that is released from the empty follicle after ovulation.

Zygote

After the egg cell has been fertilized by sperm & the cells begin to divide, this entity is no longer a sperm or ovum, it is a zygote.

Blastocyst

Also sometimes referred to as a "proembryo," this is a stage of development between zygote & embryo after conception. At this stage the fertilized egg is growing yet not attached to the uterine wall (in *implantation*).

Estrogen

A family of primary female sex hormones.

Estrogenic

Promotes production of or contains the hormone estrogen.

Oxytocic

Promotes production of or contains the hormone oxytocin.

Emmenagogue

A substance that promotes menstrual bleeding.

Abortifacient

A substance that can cause an abortion.

Nervine

A substance that is calming to the nervous system.

Qi

Lifeforce energy in Taoist & Traditional Chinese Medicine traditions.

Resources

More from Samantha Zipporah

The Conscious Contraception Skillshare

A self paced study skillshare you can access on my website, from which "Please Bleed!" is an excerpt. In this offering participants will receive information & support for creating a conscious contraception plan as unique as they are. This course integrates physiologic realities with socio-political, & psycho-spiritual dimensions of fertility. Participants will receive practical foundational biology education as well as exposure to a rich array of spiritual philosophies & practices.

This offering is for you if you want to avoid pregnancy while claiming inner authority through body sovereignty & literacy.

Mentorship Program

In depth individualized education & support for kindred spirits. Mentees receive access to all of my online courses & written materials, including works in progress, as well as live one on one sessions for counsel, care, & accountability on their path.

Patreon

Patrons receive access to my works in progress, creative writing, curated resources, Ask Me Anything sessions, discounts on my books, & more.

See samanthazipporah.com for updated description of current offerings.

Cycle Health

* *Mother Earth Embodied* Samantha Zipporah

* *Wild Power* Sjanie Wurlitzer & Alexandra Pope

* *Woman Code* Alisa Vitti

* *The Fifth Vital Sign* Lisa Jack

* *Heavy Flow* Amanda Laird

* *The Period Repair Manual* Dr. Lara Briden

Fertility Awareness Method & Contraception

* *Taking Charge of Your Fertility* Toni Weschler

* *The Garden of Fertility* Katie Singer

* *Types of Fertility Awareness Based Methods*

* *Natural Birth Control*

FAM Educators

* Ashley Hartman Annis

* The Fertility Awareness Project ~ Nathalie D

* Fertility Charting ~ Jessie Brebner

* The Cuntsultant ~ Vienna Farlow

* Cycle Wise ~ Caitlin Mcmurty

* The Well School of Body Literacy ~ Sarah Bly

* AFAP Directory of Certified Instructors

Herbal Allies for Avoiding Pregnancy

* *Natural Liberty* FREE PDF Sage Femme Collective

* *Eve's Herbs* John Riddle

* *Contraception & Abortion from the Ancient World to the Renaissance* John Riddle

* Sisterzeus.com

* *Herbal for The Childbearing Year* Susun Weed

* "Queen Anne's Lace for Fertility Management" workshop from Molly Dutton Kenny

* *Eosoma*

Sacred Sexuality

* *Mapping The Yoniverse* Samantha Zipporah

* *Desire* Daniel Odier

* *Urban Tantra* Barbara Carellas

* *The Multi-Orgasmic Woman* by Mantak Chia & Rachel Abrams

* Shakti Temple Arts ~ Jade Egg, Taoist, & Tantric teachings

* Layla Martin, Tantra

Trauma Healing, Embodiment & Sexuality

✳ Somatic Sexological Body Work

✳ *The Body Keeps The Score* Bessel van der Kolk

✳ *The Body Is Not An Apology* Sonia Renee Taylor

✳ *Come As You Are* Emily Nagoski

✳ *Vagina* Naomi Wolf

About The Author

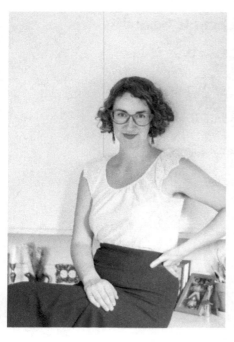

Samantha Zipporah is a practical & radical medicine woman. She is an educator, author, & activist who inspires individuals to claim their power through body literacy & sovereignty.

A former birth doula whose roots of study can be found deep in traditional midwifery "womb to tomb" style care, Sam supports her community with a full spectrum of fertility, sexuality, & pregnancy experiences. Her 20+ years of experience in service spans personal, professional, & clinical contexts. She provides vital life changing education for everyone from professionals to preteens. Her approach is grounded in a solid understanding of biochemistry & biology, & nourished by a gift for levity & depth of spirituality. Friends have joked that her business tagline should be, "If anything's going in or out of a cervix, call Sam."

Sam offers guidance & education to folks all over the world via video chat, e-books, & online courses. She also teaches live classes & retreats.

To learn more about Sam & her work please visit her at www.samanthazipporah.com

About The Illustrator

MAUREEN WALRATH

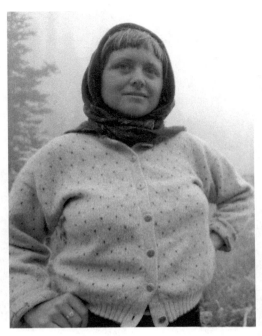

Mo is a guest on S'Klallam land in so-called rain shadowed Port Townsend, Washington where cormorants dive & eagles tell glacier memory sky stories - tending grief in baskets, bending water, shapeshifting - remembering how to be human as a white, cis woman, as a soft & fierce student of birth/death/burial/blood mysteries, reverent farmer, full spectrum doula, collaborative/interdisciplinary creatress/clown, & truth-speaking healer with ancestral lines from west coast of Ireland & Main River lands in Germany. To learn more about Mo & her amazing work see www.woventhresholds.com